T
A
C
T

Webster defines Tact as

"*: a keen sense of what to do or say in order to maintain good relations with others or avoid offense "

Written By;

Alexander Westersund

Edited by;

eldraughon (Fiver)

This book was supposed to have 52 good points; one point to conquer a week, for a solid year. But, We settled on a few less than that so you have the whole month of December off of the self improvement train to enjoy with your friends and family and focus on all your yearly accomplishments; and get geared up for another year to crush it.

"You gotta been keen to make the green!"

- **Alexander Westersund, September 2022**

Contents

This book is written for the young go getter who wants to become the best in the game. You already bought the book, so let's GO!

A common definition of the word success is the accomplishment of an aim or purpose. To make success achievable, think of what you can do, what is within your control, and aim towards that goal. Once your aim is zeroed in on a target, you might not get a bullseye every time, but you will hit the main target. That's 90% of the game in life, hit your target and spend your free time working on your accuracy. Think of it this way; you do not have to hit a home run to get to home plate. Work your way around the bases to the best of YOUR ability. Count your wins even when they seem insignificant. Remember: not everyday is a playoff tournament. We gotta show up to practice first.

And that's the goal of this book: To help you to help you show up and practice which will lead you to success in life.

The content you are about to read is geared for the younger crowd who wants to get started on the right path in life. You might not even realize you are on a path, but we all are. The path we choose and follow early in life will plot our course. Once you are over the hill; motivation, drive, and encouragement from others goes into massive decline. Family and friends start dying, no one wants to get physical, sex drive is decreased, cognitive ability goes down, testosterone starts dropping about 1% a year, and once available partners are now out of the dating pool, has kids, or is obese. Possibly all three.

You can read this book point by point, back to front or front to back, but I hope you highlight the ideas you like and come to realize that if you just aim at something you will be miles ahead of the rest.

There's something in this book for everyone. Even if you only take away one sentence, just a tiny part of one point, you are further ahead than before you started. When you start to free your mind of toxic thoughts, you'll have **more mental real estate to grow your vision.**

This is not a book in the traditional sense. It's more of a guide to help you onto the path of enlightenment of a better life, for YOU. To have a crystal-clear vision we must understand what is on the other side of enlightenment. Some of you have been there and know it can be full of despair, resentment, anger, malevolence, and frustration. But if you allow this book to be a mentor, you can avoid regression and keep heading down the path of progression. There is no such thing as being in-between. You're either progressing towards positivity and the life you want to live, or you are regressing. Once you switch from negative to positive, you be unstoppable. Let's get started.

Moving Beyond Boomer Advice

When I left high school at 18, most of the information and guidance provided was from baby boomers. Now, at 37, after going through three economic downturns (2008, 2015, and now COVID 2020), we realize much of what is wrong with the boomer mentality and how boomers did things that benefited them and no one else. They were the first generation to have an easy life, everyone blames the millennials for feeling entitled, but where did that originate from? BOOMERS. (Sorry, this book is not for you if you were born between 1946- 1964).

Boomers definitely failed to plan for retirement. According to the 19th Annual Retirement Survey of Workers conducted by the TransAmerica Center for Retirement Studies, boomers have only saved $152,000 (USD) for retirement. Not nearly enough. Who will pick up the slack? Future generations will be taxed to pay the bills of our aging seniors. This has forced the left side of the government to become more radically socialist, increasing taxes, reforms on everything, and suppressing the capitalistic ideals that drive small businesses to succeed. The right, on the other hand, sometimes responds too strongly the other way with tax cuts, cutting government pensions, removing government jobs, and trying to balance the checkbook after the left has overspent. Now the boomer generation who did not save is stuck, and the younger crowd is stuck with the bill.

This book is designed to get past the archaic advice of earlier generations. It is a revised edition of tips and tricks to push you to the next level. It is geared toward the long view and is an easy-to-read guide for you to utilize as you work to hit your goals and jump over the landmines in the game of life that your homeroom teacher neglected to mention.

Now future generations must step up their game to win. We have been presented with a tough, uphill battle, left to deal directly with the past generation. This is not a slag on the boomer generation. Rather, it is a guide to encourage up and comers that life is not all doom and gloom. Just because things have been done a certain way for a long time does not negate the fact that there is always room for improvement. Sometimes the older generations will dispute this because they've been hardened in their ways.

I think my peers would agree that many boomers were of the "Do as I say not as I do" mentality. They had some rebellion and resentment in their blood from being raised by a tough generation who had to endure the great depression but never endured the adversity that led the older generation to greatness in mind, body and spirit. Now, once again, the current generation is faced with overwhelming challenges that we need to face together. We need to get rid of the 'what bout me mentality' and think about the next guy or gal in the trades. We like to say, "If you see it, you own it."

Time to step up to the plate and hit a home run.

Four Foundational Things to Remember

There are four things I find important to keep front and center in my mind.

- Buying Choices
- Health Choices
- Sustainable Choices
- Societal Choices

On buying choices:

We must all be cognizant of the ever-changing world and seek out sustainable solutions for complex problems. One of them is the lack of quality in manufactured items. The last thing we need or want to do is waste our hard-earned money on things that keep costing us money. When we spend our after-tax cash money, we expect to get something for it, and we expect those things to last. That's why it's so frustrating to waste money at Walmart on the Chinese garbage they stock the shelves with that do nothing to benefit our local economy. When I was a child, you could buy many high-quality products produced in either Canada or the USA that would last for 5-10 years, or longer, instead of the one or two or few years things last now. Part of this problem is because boomers wanted things for cheaper, so they sent all our manufacturing over to China. Garbage is what we get back.

On health choices:

Another problem is the obesity crisis. During the 60s there was a bit of a movement that started this crisis, and everyone needs to be aware of what it is. Massive amounts of sugar were added to breakfast cereals and the consumption of pop/soda went through the roof. Then in the 70s high fructose corn syrup (HFCS) replaced sugar in sodas and really screwed us up. Now HFCS is disguised as Sugar/Glucose-Fructose. Here is a taste test, try Mexican Coke which is now available in Canada and the USA and compare it to Canadian/American coke. Mexican coke is much better tasting, and one could argue healthier. HFCS has been shown to increase insulin resistance, diabetes, and other health problems when compared to regular sugar. HFCS is made from cornstarch. Corn is one of the most widely known GMO foods on the planet. Humans cannot digest corn by the way. The point of all this is that we need to be accountable in our actions when sourcing out the cheapest alternative. That is why HFCS was invented. It was a cheap, liquid alternative to cane and beet sugar. The consumers and government at the time allowed this. They did not consider the repercussions of this unhealthy sugar alternative.

On sustainable choices:

Many of our future successes will be based on our choices of today. We must make sustainable, long-term choices that do not nickel and dime us to death. Life quality has increased dramatically over the past 20 years and so has the cost of living. Without a two income house hold, living in major cities is hard; but this book is designed to set you up so if you put in the time now when you are fit and able, you will be able to mold your lifestyle to become fulfilling and fruitful without having to sacrifice to the point of being a minimalist (although that works for some people).

On societal choices:

One of the best and most fulfilling things you can do in your life is to serve others. But before you can serve others, your must satisfy your own needs. This book will help build you up by tweaking your day-to-day mindset to shift from negative to positive. From I can't to I already did that before sunup. Not only will consistently making these types of choices improve *your* life, when you turn your focus outward to help and serve others, you will be a model to them and potentially turn their life around, as well.

As mentioned before, this book does not need to be read in any particular order. Each point is adaptable to every reader's personality. Take what you want, leave what you do not want. If you are looking for success in life you will never find it. Success is elusive, it is always right around the corner. But, once you tick off all the boxes and lead by example, you will be amazed how quickly success finds you.

Keep reading to discover the tips and tricks that will level up your life.

Start Your Day Right

Socrates said the only thing that makes one man different from another, is his habits. (Man / Woman / Person/ Alien) The best way to start your day right is with a solid MORNING ROUTINE. If you do not read any other tip in this book, read this, and then burn the book.

To start your day right, create a sustainable morning routine and stick to it. One thousand push-ups every morning is not sustainable, but 25 is.

Starting your day off right begins the night before with getting a good night's sleep and waking up in a positive way. So, let's talk about the things that can interfere with getting a good night's sleep. Two things are: what you put in your body before you go to sleep, and what you use to wake up in the morning.

Go to bed with a fairly empty stomach. Digestion uses a lot of energy and blood, and when we sleep, we want to maximize our brain blood flow. Proper blood flow to the brain allows us to sleep better and enter REM sleep faster.

Also, avoid alcohol at all costs before bedtime. Not only does alcohol delay digestion, it reduces our body's ability to absorb water. Alcohol can really mess with your sleep. It might make you sleepy, but that does not last unless you get really hammered. Then you can have an old-fashioned hangover the next day. A hangover is not just a headache. Alcohol is a powerful drug and too much of it can cause dehydration, poor sleep quality, and can cause long-term health problems.

When I go to bed with a fairly empty stomach and get a good night's sleep, I find I wake up just before the alarm goes off, so I avoid that negative feeling associated with a buzz or some other sound intended to get me out of bed.

If you don't want to use an alarm clock because of the glare or noise, use a cell phone or watch since they offer a choice of ringtones and aren't quick as jarring as the sound of an alarm clock. Here is a photo of a watch shipped directly to my door off eBay. I am hard on equipment, but it has been over a year since I've had this bad boy and there are no signs of wear. If I buy a "Guess" branded watch, guess what? It comes from China. So, in some circumstances, buying off eBay, Amazon, or similar makes sense, as in Canada I cannot buy a Canadian made watch of similar quality for less than $100. I would rather spend the money I save supporting local growers and farmers.

Once you manage what you put into your body before going to bed so you can get a good night's sleep, and you've got an alarm that wakes you gently, you can move on to your morning routine. Do not try to establish a successful morning routine before you get your night routine down. Once you have practiced your night routine successfully for a few weeks, start thinking of how you are going to win by sticking to your morning routing MOST mornings.

MOST mornings is achievable. EVERY morning is not. There will be mornings when you feel sick, or you are tired after a restless night. Sometimes you won't have time or be too stressed out and just need a day off. That's okay! We are not robots. So even if we only do our morning routine 51% of the time, we are still progressing. If you slip to 49%, shame on you. That's regressing.

If you cannot form a simple morning routine for most mornings, burn this book and fall in line with the average person who is not self aware, does not care about his fellow man, and just wants to do the minimum that socialists love. If you have that extra 1% in you, read on. I do not hate socialism by the way, there are some really good points a socialist argues for and I'd agree with them. But there is a reason why the USSR dissolved. Look at Czechoslovakia, a socialist nation. Once they broke away from the USSR the country went through massive changes, become more of a social free market, and is a popular tourist destination that attracts millions each year.

Buying your first car

Before you even start looking, I suggest watching a few videos on YouTube. There is one old cat I love to follow, Scotty Kilmer. While I don't agree with his hap hazard attitude at all times, he has some good points. Toyota is a reliable brand. Never buy a new vehicle since they depreciate up to 30% when you drive them off the lot.)

The number one thing to do if you are not going to do ANYTHING else is to get it inspected from an honest and reputable mechanic before you buy. Have compression and leak down tests performed. This tells the mechanic how well important parts of the engine like the valves and pistons are performing. Replacing these parts can be expensive. Have the mechanic note the colors of the fluids, especially the transmission fluid. If it is brown, walk away. It's supposed to be red. If it is brown, damage has occurred. No matter how much you like the vehicle, if these tests return poor results, you are in for costly repairs. If the inspection checks out and the car has two fobs, no damage history, and all the maintenance history is provided, you are on the right track. Avoid buying from a wholesale dealer and at all costs, don't buy at an auction. Try to buy a Honda or Toyota. If you can drive a stick shift, go that route, it might even be cheaper. The only downside to a stick shift is that many people cannot drive them anymore. Honda just stopped making them in their Accord.

The only downside to some Toyotas and Hondas is they need specific maintenance done to prevent big problems later. This relates directly to the timing belts. If these belts are not changed at their required intervals, the belt may snap and damage the engine. When replacing the timing belt, it is a no brainer to also replace the water pump and associated components like idler, tensioner and seals. These parts are typically included in the kit. The same with replacing a clutch, do the whole kit at the same time. Things like this blow me away. Often you can order a specific part when fixing a component on a car, but order the "kit" or ask if it is available since it is usually around the same price and lets you address all the issues relating to the failure.

Eating Healthy

Yes, we all know we have to eat our vegetables but with obesity almost cresting 50% in North America this is more important than ever. You do not want to be the richest guy or gal in the graveyard.

When thinking about eating healthy, the easiest way to transition to a healthy lifestyle is to not count calories, do intermittent fasting, or try nutrient timing. It is very easy. Look at what our ancestors ate and try to replicate that diet. Limit processed foods. Eat, good quality meat, wild game is the best if possible.

The easiest way to do eat healthy is to just track your macros. For most men it is suggested 1g / lb of LEAN body weight. Say you are 200 lbs, 20% body fat. You do not need to eat 200 grams of protein. You should shoot for about 160 grams if you are working out hard, about half that if you are just trying to maintain a healthy weight.

Hot tip: all bison is grass fed. A friend of mine says the beef he raises that is grass fed tastes better and has a better fat composition. Once you start eating more of the good stuff, you will automatically eat less of the bad stuff. Once you start eating right you can move on to the next tip about working out. All the trendy stuff like keto, IF, nutrient timing, special vitamins and so forth can be experimented with once you are getting your 5-10 vegetable servings in per day, drinking 8 glasses of water a day, have cut out all soda/pop (if you are in Canada), quit smoking, and limited your alcohol consumption to one drink a day max) no binge drinking!

To summarize, stay on your goals. A little tip that is easy to incorporate to keep your weight in check is to consume a little apple cider vinegar each day. ACV has been shown in peer reviewed studies to balance blood sugar and trim the waistline. Downside? It tastes nasty. But if you take a big jug of water, put in some fresh-squeezed organic lemon juice with some turmeric for increased anti-inflammatory action with a couple big squirts of ACV, it isn't too bad. And it helps alkalize your body which some theorize makes it more difficult for cancer cells to grow and replicate.

Work Out Often

How often, how hard, and how long? Studies have shown more than 45 minutes of intense training raises cortisol levels. This means after 45 minutes you could be doing more harm then good. So what? Well, you are trying to reduce cortisol (stress) by working out. You do not want to be increasing it. So, after 45 minutes to an hour, pack it in. Do some stretches. Take a sauna if you can, followed by an ice old shower and a protein shake and you are off to having a great start to your day.

The best time of day to work out is early morning. The fasted state is the best as your glycogen stores will be at their lowest and will help eradicate fat in the most efficient way possible. Typically, a good pre-workout is not some chemical concoction with unknown amounts of chemicals, but two shots of espresso with MCT oil does wonders. The MCT oil, typically derived from coconuts, gets burned as energy and is not stored as fat. MCT oil has been around on the supplement store shelves for over 30 years. There is a theory when you mix the MCT oil in with the coffee it helps regulate the caffeine uptake as your gallbladder needs to release bile to digest the fat and this can take some time, so you get a nice slow rise in blood stream caffeine levels and slow drop off, not the typical crash and burn effect. Not sure if this is true, but it is a good theory.

Healthy fats are the hardest thing to incorporate in the diet; so, to reiterate on point number two, try and hit your daily macro fat intake. I do not try to have a macro goal on carbs. Once I hit my macro goals on fat and protein, I top up my fuel tank with some complex carbs and can maintain my body weight with ease. The main take away… don't overdo it.

There was a body builder in the 80s who had one training session once a week that was a long session. I would advise to train every other day. On days you train, make sure to hit your Marcos, have a protein shake after every session, and avoid alcohol at all costs. Alcohol is great, but for every pleasure you pay for it in pain. The problem with alcohol is three-fold. If you have calories in your system, your body prioritizes to digest the alcohol first, which is very taxing on your liver. Then, once the alcohol is digested and your metabolism is slowed down, the remaining calories will be digested. The alcohol has probably disturbed your gut bacteria so you will likely not get all the nutrients out of the food you had previously ingested which leads to empty calories being stored as, yup. I don't have to finish that because I know you're smart enough to figure it out.

Music

Music is the key to relaxation and motivation. Try to get a few hours of music in daily. It helps motivate, boosts mood, and promotes relaxation. If you really want to take it up a notch, check out binaural beats on YouTube. This type of music has been shown to enhance sleep quality and can be used to help with relaxation.

When I say music, I am not talking about the radio. The radio can poison your wellbeing with talk of politics and other current events that do not apply to you upping your game. When you are in your car, hit your Bluetooth from your cell to disconnect and relax while driving. If you don't know where to start, Spotify is great. If you're on a road trip and need to stream some music, check out sonicweb. It's a cheap app that lets you download music to your phone at only a one-time cost. Blows all the monthly mandated music subscription services out of the water. I think I bought it for $3.99 5 years ago. Nice thing is you can download it on WiFi and then just listen as you cruise.

Sleep

When it comes to sleep, it's quality over quantity. Try and stick with 7.5-8.5 hours per night. Any more or less reduces performance. Sleep is like a drug, the more you get the more you need, so make sure to be strict and never go over 9 hours unless you are recovering from a surgery or sickness. If you find yourself tired and you're still sleeping soundly for over 8.5 hours per night, go to the doctor and get your hormone and iron levels checked. These can have a major impact on your well-being.

Continuity and congruency are key when hitting sleep targets. Going to bed at the same time every night (even on weekends) and not oversleeping is key to a healthy lifestyle. Keep your caffeine and stimulant consumption limited to morning. Alcohol should be avoided three hours prior to bed. Alcohol can have nasty effects on sleep and should be limited if not eradicated.

Moving Out and Up

Eventually you will need to move out of your parents' house and get your own pad. This sounds easy, but there are a few hoops you need to go through. One hidden expense is the damage deposit. Make sure when you sign your lease you get a copy and it in writing. Best is to video tape your initial walk through, make notes, and get your landlord to sign that everyone agrees to the terms and conditions. Going to court mediation to get your damage deposit back is not fun, and typically courts like to rule in the landlord's favor. The number of bad tenants in the world outweighs the good or we wouldn't need all the regulations we have adopted.

When you are getting cable set up, make sure you negotiate and negotiate hard. Avoid signing contracts and be wary of the promos they offer which often come with hidden strings and stipulations attached. Each state and province have their own rental rules that should be followed to the best of your ability. When you move out, make sure you give 30 days notice and record your move out inspection in case your landlord turns into a slumlord and wants to pocket your damage deposit dollars.

Efficiency

Be ruthless with your time. If someone in your circle isn't bringing all they have to the table and contributing in a positive manner, just tell them you can do better. If they don't get it, move on. As an automation technician by trade (that's automation not automotive), we make efficiency happen. We do not have time for down time. We do not have time for excuses. We want things to work, and when they don't, we have our system set up to send an alarm. Set your life up like this and program your mind in a way to alert you when things are moving along as quickly and effectively as possible.

This is subconscious training. You do not want to waste the brain power of your conscious mind to pick up on this. It is theorized that your sub conscious mind is 100 times stronger than your conscious mind. Like the great plagiarist Thomas Edison said, "Never go to bed without a request to your subconscious mind." My takeaway is that someone smart enough to manipulate Nikola Tesla is someone worth listening to. Before you go to sleep, think of something you want to do, progress in, or enhance. Then ask your subconscious mind, or better yet, instruct your mind to work on this problem while you sleep. For example, if you want a 6-pack, simply ask in your head before you pass out, what can I do in my life to help achieve my goal of getting 6-pack abs. And keep asking yourself. Eventually, when you are picking up that doughnut on your coffee break you will either drop it, or no longer want it because your subconscious directive will kick in. It's like a mild state of hypnosis that you control.

Making Contacts

Making contacts, networking, making and keeping friends. You are who you hang with. You are a blend of your five closest contacts, so pick ones who will stick around. Now when it comes to meeting people and connecting, it seems as though Facebook, Instagram, Snap Chat, Tik Tok and all the other social medial platforms are the way to go. Are they? What are you benefiting besides depleting your dopamine levels? Especially when those apps can breach your data. Not cool. The people who really matter in your life will follow you outside of your social media.

To create a growing circle that matters, try and send out as many birthday cards and greeting cards and congrats cards as possible. If you send one card a week, that's 52 cards in a year. If you get the cards at the dollar store, that's only $52 at $1 per card. That is a small price to show people who you are, that you are caring and considerate of others. It is scientifically proven that the more conscientious a person is, naturally, the less anxiety they are shown to have. Connecting with 52 people in one year via old snail mail has a massive impact over the 500 friends on Facebook you seldom connect with. Check this out: when you meet a new person, instead of saying nice to meet you… see you later, finish up with this line:

"It was good or "GREAT" to meet someone as interesting as you. Can I get your contact information so I know how to get in touch with you?"

And then to put the icing on the cake, mention to them your sign and ask them for theirs. I've never had a person decline. Once that bridge has been crossed, it's mighty fine to tell them your birthday because 99% of the time they will hit you back with theirs. The year is not important. Once you glean this info, put a yearly reminder for their birthday in your cell, and have it remind you one day before their birthday. Then, one day before their birthday, give them a buzz and say:

"Hey, your birthday is coming up tomorrow. Any plans?"

Works wonders. Once you have built up your network of like-minded individuals you have one last thing to do. DO NOT lose your contact list. Find an app you like, grab the VCF virtual contact file, and back it up, email it to yourself and in the subject line tag it "Contact List". If your phone ever goes AWOL you have a direct link to your contacts. This ensures you will always have your black book up to date and on point. ICloud is great, but not 100% reliable.

Oh, and the last but most important tip. If you meet someone and you get along well but they do one, two, or three things that annoy you, but you don't want to tell them and risk your friendship, do it anyway. Tell them. If you don't, you will subconsciously sabotage the friendship by seeking retribution for the annoyance. Every action has an equal and opposite... well, you get the point if you made it this far.

Networking is one of the most important things a young person can do to level up, whether it is romantically, socially, or economically.

Stress

Stress is a sex killer, motivational killer, and sleep killer. Once all these three massive, important factors are crushed, it can really affect your well being and your drive to thrive. Stress is an important motivational factor in life, but it must be managed. Once you are over stressed, it's too late. You have to take care of yourself and hit the eject button long before you have a meltdown. People can become bi-polar (a chemical change in the brain) from being over stressed and often this change is permanent.

The only way your body can excrete the stress hormone, cortisol, is through perspiration. Exercise not your thing? Try a sauna, the traditional way followed by immersion in ice cold water. Repeat three times for best effect. Infrared saunas will suffice, but do not get hot enough. To really amp up the cleansing, try and find a sauna where you can pour water on the rocks. If you cannot do a sauna, throw on a garbage bag or rain jacket and climb some stairs or go for a walk. That will force your body to sweat and, quick. Doesn't take long. A good cleanse followed by a cold shower should help you snap out of the danger zone.

At all costs, avoid going to your doctor to get medication. Often the medication is addictive and only works for a short time before you need to increase dosage. I recommend HTP-5 as a natural stress reliver, as well St. Johns Wort which has a lot of beneficial stress reliving benefits. St. Johns Wort is the most widely prescribed anti-depressant in Germany, the most technologically advanced country in the world. Webber Naturals is my go-to brand for these products. I first read about Kava-Kava in Arnold's *Pumping Iron* book and tried it. It works, but I think there are better and healthier alternatives as there are some toxicity reports associated with Kava-Kava.

Try and get in a daily routine that involves some meditation and limit your screen time an hour before bed. Try journaling or at least reflect on your day about what was good. Incorporating the flow of positive thoughts helps build new neural pathways for the endorphins to flow on when you do get excited about something good in your life. This can be addictive. Try and batch when you use your phone or email. Instead of checking your email or Facebook every five minutes, schedule time to use your devices. When we get text messages, we get a strong dopamine (feel good hormone). Depleted your dopamine store makes you feel drained.

Last tip. Avoid excessive alcohol consumption. Any more than one drink a day is over doing it and can promote alcoholism. Let's avoid that path. One glass of red wine here and there can have some benefits. but be careful with how big your glass is.

Religion

It is good to have faith in something. If we don't believe in anything external, we won't be open enough to believe in anything internal. As the most evolved creature on planet earth (that we know of), we need to continue to evolve and become better. Some people need that higher guidance in their lives and find it in different ways to include spiritualism and religious beliefs. I would like to imagine all religions should be accepted as everyone should be entitled to their beliefs. One can be religious but not spiritual, spiritual, but not religious, but the enlightened and inquisitive mind will be most satisfied when open to both. Albert Einstein said, "Science without Religion is lame, Religion without Science is blind." Mr. Einstein was not atheist, but Agnostic.

Credit

Everyone needs it at some point in time. The higher your credit score, the easier it is to buy a car, house, or even a TV when you want to use plastic or someone else's capital to make a big purchase. As soon as you are able, get a bank account in your name, as well as a social security number. Once these two are up and running, you are building credit. Having a simple cellphone bill coming in once a month and paying the bill on time, every time, is all it takes to start getting your FICO score close to that 900 range. Anywhere over 800 is considered excellent. The lower your number, the more difficult it will be to negotiate a good rate or even get a loan from some lenders without collateral or a co-signer. You want to be on your own; not tied up with a co-signer who could manipulate you.

Hobbies

You need down time, It's mandatory for humans as if we can't unwind, it hurts our sleep, workouts, eating habits and more. Prevents cabin fever. Let's our thoughts and body interact and helps us enter flow state. A lot of our relaxation does not come when we are sleeping. Feel good hormones start flowing when we are doing something we are passionate about. When endorphins flow, time flies by, and more feel-good chemicals are produced. This is a positive feedback loop. When in the flow state, time will fly by, and a sense of wellbeing will be felt in your soul.

Endocrine Disruptors

Avoid endocrine disruptors at all costs as they will really screw you over; and not just you, they can affect your kids, too. These little gremlins are cumulative. They lead to bad things: birth defects, tumors, and cancer are a few of the nasties you will be left with. Heating food in a plastic container in the microwave will promote endocrine disruption. BPA free water bottles are now popular, but we recommend stainless steel. Not aluminum another endocrine disruptor. Phytoestrogens are endocrine disruptors, particularly soy, which is extremely bad for men as it promotes estrogen!

Cigarette smoke is an endocrine disruptor. Many things that are endocrine disruptors are also known carcinogens. Alcohol. Prime example. See where this is going. AVOID AVOID AVOID. Engage yourself in learning what really is 'good' for you. Just because everyone does something and it is common practice doesn't mean it is right or good for you. Fluoride is such an outdated additive to our water and toothpaste. "Fluoride reduces tooth decay" may have been true 50 years ago when we didn't have the fancy toothbrushes of today, and where we didn't go to the dentist every six months. Fluoride has been clinically shown to lower sperm count. 97% of Western Europe does not fluoridate their water. I am a little biased myself as I had fluoride as a child and now suffer from fluorosis where my tooth enamel has been adversely affected. Fluoride can get absorbed very fast through your gumline and then go straight to your blood stream, get filtered through the kidneys and then adsorbed into your bones (think chewing tobacco here and how quickly you get a buzz when you stick that nasty stuff in your teeth). Fluoride can get adsorbed into your bones. Avoid fluoride and try and limit endocrine disruption from happening in your body. Do not participate in poisoning your body. Fluoride is just one example that we can all cut out immediately.

The Power of the Subconscious

Most of our day-to-day doings are controlled by our subconscious. We don't need to think while doing many activities as these processes are partially handled by the subconscious. Driving, brushing your teeth, waking up at the same time every day, saying "hello" when you answer the phone, are things you do not have to always consciously be aware of. Your subconscious can help you out.

If we can start making requests of our subconscious mind, our daily tasks will be easier. Say you see something and want to remember what you saw, you consciously tell your mind that you want to remember this. Make an effort to remember it and your subconscious mind will do the rest. The more you practice this the easier it becomes.

Jose Silvia has written an excellent book on this called *The Silva Mind Control Method*. Meditation and proper relaxation techniques will assist in this. Binaural beats can help. If you have ever been to a hypnotist, you can see the results for yourself. Recommend checking out the Wim Hof Method. Very similar to the Sylvia method. Both are good, but the Wim Hof is a little more up to date. His audio book from the library was excellent with over 8 CDs. Wim hof has shown he has control over his Vagus nerve. Wow.

Accountability

When we are accountable to ourselves, we let the BS wash over ourselves and not stick. We become invincible, and the only way to acquire this trait is to hold yourself accountable 100% of the time. If you see it, own it. It can be hard to do when you see everyone slacking and just being mindless. Live in the moment. When someone gets in your face with anxiety about future tasks and is living in their heads, use Vin Diesel's line, "I live my life a quarter mile at a time, and in those 10 seconds or less, nothing else matters." That will snap them back to reality.

Communication

It's free. Learn to use it, work on it, and follow up promptly. Going to a meeting? Before the meeting send an email that you will be there early if anyone has any questions. Bring coffee to grease the wheels. Got a job interview? Send a follow up thank you card. Not heard back from a client? Break the ego and reach out. Be the better person and set an example! Let others know you are approachable and willing to put in the work to make it happen. Most of our communication in person is non-verbal and body language is huge; but with cell phones, computers, and electronics, we know we must use our words. Texting has cut out one important tool we use for communication, tonality, and often a simple text can be misinterpreted. Avoid the one-word responses and sign emails with words like cordially, truthfully, honestly, and other feel-good terms to ensure a positive reply.

Often, people in upper management get to these roles and neglect others below them. This decreases respect and enables contempt to brew. STOP IT and get real. Often the quiet types are the ones that know. Sometimes the introverted crowds are the people you need to drill into and get them engaged. It's interesting to note that most CIOs in the world are introverts. Barrack Obama, introvert. Einstein? Introvert. And both of them are Nobel Prize winners. Sometimes the quiet ones are the ones you need on your team, and often introverts are so in 'their head' they pick up on non-verbal communication like nobody's business as they are paying close attention to everything. If you can connect to them on their higher level, you can stack those wins for your team.

Be Ruthless Who You Associate With

It's better to fly solo than fly in a group that's going to crash and burn. If your friends and acquaintances do not challenge and engage you; look elsewhere. You are the company you keep. Like Gordon Gekko said, "It's not always the most popular guy that gets the job done." Be the non popular guy. Get the job done. If all your friends want to do is have a good time and not set any goals, you need new friends. Find a group that pushes you to be better and stay motivated. Usually, friends like this aren't found at the bar, but at the ski hill, gym, church, or school. If you hang out with winners, you will become a winner. If you hang out with losers, you might not be the top loser, but you will end up somewhere in the middle of the pack. Wolves don't put up with losers and neither should you. We are most closely related to wolves than any other species.

Get a Magnetic Bracelet

A magnetic bracelet helps massively with sleep quality. I bought one on sale for three bucks. Tried it. No longer do I have to take Melatonin. The brand I recommend is Sabona. They have been making these things for 50 years. Lots of theory behind these bracelets, but from my experience, it doesn't cost you anything to wear it once you buy one. I saw them for 20 bucks on Amazon. There have been studies that shows evidence that these bracelets boost melatonin levels. There is also some theory that it helps circulation. Many people say that after six months, it still looks and feels new.

Quick Tips

- The stock market has three major indexes: DOW, NASDAQ, and S&P 500. Each one specializes in a different area. Diversification in all is your best bet to weather a downturn.
- kPA to psi, divide or times by 7.
- -40 C is -40 F. 32 F is 0 Deg C. C. Very useful as 400 millions of people still use Fahrenheit.
- You can contribute to your Retirement Savings Plan until the last day of February for last year's taxes, (Canada)
- Calories in does not equal calories out.
- Your brain uses a lot of calories
- Testosterone is highest in the morning as is cortisol, which motivates you to get out of bed.
- Intermittent fasting can help high blood sugar fat loss.
- Rats have shown to repair DNA in fasted states, and there is speculation this is true in humans.
- Start a trading account as soon as you turn 18. Avoid Robin Hood. Crypto is risky.
- Try and plant a few trees every year.
- Eat organic honey that is non-pasteurized (RAW) the only food that never expires

Cookware

Is cookware all the same? After spending thousands of dollars on cookware and living through the Teflon crisis and the transition away from carcinogenic coated pans, we should be able to agree that there are a few healthy, non-toxic options. Buy high-end ceramic cookware or use cast iron. Do not use old, scratched pans. You do not know their history! Cast Iron will last forever but can be tricky to cook with. If you buy cheap Teflon (PFOA, C8, the harmful chemical in Teflon) coated pans, the coating can scratch and chip and then you may ingest it. These pans are no longer sold in North America, but why risk it. Avoid Teflon pans at all costs. Find a pan you like with a ceramic coating that is guaranteed not to chip or flake. This will transition into my next topic.

Clothing

In 2021 we go through clothes like the ones we are wearing are on fire. Now we are in the age we have to realize purchasing and repurchasing clothing hurts not only our bottom line. The environment is being directly impacted as well. According to the Institute of Sustainable Communication, the clothing industry is the second-**highest polluter** of clean water. Buying cheap, throw away clothes from your favorite stores like H and M, Urban Outfitters, and Army and Navy are suspected as being part of these numbers. Look for high quality clothing that will last a long time. I personally like Mountain Equipment Co-Op (MEC) in Canada. We find most of our clothing bought here does not wear out, fade, rip or shrink. Better yet, you can often buy tax free almost new clothing at the Salvation Army, and sometimes make a couple bucks flipping some for a profit.

Condom Usage

Not as easy as it sounds. The most important financial responsibility anyone can easily do is stay baby free until you're married. Having a child before marriage with a girl friend or random other, or you as a woman popping out a child at a young age will destroy most of your future opportunities. There are exceptions, but we are talking about statistical probabilities in this book. You can still make it in life. I am not anti-child. I am anti-child when you are not ready. The number one thing a man can do to prevent a child is to wear a rubber that is within its expiration date! Learning how to put it on is one thing, there is a right and wrong way, so you have a 50/50 chance of getting it right. The other thing is, do not think the condom won't break on you. They break, and break often, especially if lubrication is a problem. So, buy the lubricated ones. The spermicidal lubricant may be overkill, and I do not wish the feeling of spermicide going inside the urethra on any man. When ejaculating, try to pull out and ejaculate in the condom while the penis is not in the vagina. If the condom breaks and you ejaculate while inside the vagina, all the safe sex practices in the world won't save you. If you are in full stroke, you won't realize the condom broke. That 10 seconds of pleasure is not worth the lifetime of pain if you didn't want that kid!

Build Your Brand

Not on Facebook, unless it's a common interest group. Facebook friends are not your real friends. Find followers that you share common interest with. My preference is YouTube. It has much less drama than Facebook and people will subscribe your channel. Then you can monetize it. Another no brainer. Twitter, Instagram, and other platforms are all right too. YouTube has been around the longest and probably will be around long after the others fizzle. Build that subscriber base!

Sunglasses and Mineral-based Sunscreen

The sun will age you just about as fast as smoking. Protect your eyes, wear a hat, and use sunscreen if you are fair skinned. This is a priority. Fair-skinned, light-eyed people are genetically modified to adsorb more sunlight to help process more vitamin D. Keep that in mind if you're a ginger. These people are typically genetically modified by nature for Scandinavian countries but were transplanted elsewhere throughout the world and now need to be cognizant that their mutation is working against them. Black people get less skin cancer by the way. Try and wear dark, UV certified sunglasses There is minor speculation that you adsorb vitamin D through your eyes. This could be true, so I encourage people in northern climates to supplement with Vitamin D as most people some VDD (Vitamin D deficiency). It is probably more common than ADD, which has increased exponentially over the years, and interestingly, ADD can be combated with vitamin D. Did I need to put that in there? No, but if you have a hard time focusing, try vitamin D, and throw in some fish oil, and dial back your coffee intake, especially later in the day.

Vitamin D

Most people are Vitamin D deficient. Why? Probably because we aren't getting it from the sun anymore. Sunscreen, working indoors, cars, air conditioning, etc. Twenty minutes a day of sunlight is about all you need. You get thousands of units of vitamin D from the sun. If that doesn't work for you, look at Vitamin D drops. Vitamin D is not a vitamin, but a hormone, and needs to be respected as such. IF you do not get this simple hormone and are deficient, it can lead to weakened immune response, lethargy, poor calcium absorption, and seasonal depression. Vitamin D supplementation is a nominal cost, and there are no negative side effects. I highly recommend giving your favorite morning drink a squirt of Vit-D. The cheapest source I found was London Drugs Vitamin D drops. The capsules work too, but you must take a lot. Studies have found even after months of supplementation; people are still vitamin D deficient.

Checklists

Pilots use them, astronauts use them, nuclear launch personnel use them. If you want to be well organized and save money at the same time, use a checklist you can keep on your phone or a physical copy with you, while trying to accomplish certain tasks. The easiest checklist would be a grocery list. My favorite checklist is for travelling, example below. We always used to end up forgetting one thing or another, but with the checklist, you tend to have a better trip with fewer interruptions and more enjoyment while on vacation.

- travel pillow

- noise cancelling headphones

- minimum 1 Liter water bottle to fill at airport after security

- power bank (2 would be ideal)

- Snacks (nuts, tuna, fruit is good as long as you ditch it if you're going over borders)

- eye mask

- travel adapter

- charging cable for iPad and cell phone

- note pad and pen

- gum

- ear plugs

Cell Phone Usage

Scientists say cell phone usage does not promote cancer and the radiation is non-ionizing. Fact: Brain cancer has increased with increased cell phone usage. Get a Bluetooth or use a speaker phone. As well, lower sperm counts have been found with men who keep their cell in their front pocket. Some speculate it's the heat that brings on lower sperm counts, but why risk it; especially with many couples experiencing fertility issues now a days. Use an arm band or store your phone elsewhere. Airplane mode works too.

Personal Water Consumption

Eight glasses a day? Bottled? Tap? Does it matter? If you live in a big, industrialized city, chances are they fluoridate your drinking water as well as chlorinate it. More chemicals you don't need. Lead and heavy metals come from stagnant water absorbing harmful chemicals from the pipes. My old man who was a pharmacist used to praise distilled water but changed his tune to reverse osmosis. If you are doing a detox, I think distilled is the way to go for a short time, but the theory is that it has zero minerals in it and it can leech those minerals from your body if you drink too much of it. Walmart sells a distilled water with minerals added back to it for about 2 bucks CAD. I think if you have the time money and patience, get reverse osmosis water delivered and that would be the most health conscious, efficient solution.

For home filtration systems for the average person on a budget, I have read the reviews and was most impressed by the Zero Water filtration system. At around 30 bucks, I saw that during an evaluation after going through the filter, there was ZERO dissolved solids. Pretty good I'd say. You can also check the inline filters that go under your sink. Read you community water report, though, and educate yourself on what is in the water.

Eight glasses a day may be too much. If your urine is consistently clear with no hint of yellow, you may be over hydrating. Eight glasses a day is for active people, and that includes other sources of hydration like veggies and fruit. Chances are, your quantity is good, but double check your quality. Some truth behind the benefits of alkaline water. You can alkaline water by adding lemons (Yes, lemons are acidic, but in your body it turns alkaline).

Side Hustle

No matter what you do for work, try to have a side job that is usually tax free and fun. Back in 2005 I started brand building on eBay by collecting positive feedback. I only use eBay for fun, and do not consider myself a professional seller. I was blown away in 2021 how many people only use Amazon but neglect to realize many things from eBay can get ordered from China for a small fraction of the cost on Amazon, and often for free shipping. This is just an easy example.

Side hustles can be anything from cleaning cars to reviewing restaurants on your YouTube channel, to running errands or doing odd jobs for cash. Whatever your side job is, make it pay for your vacations or something to bring you joy. Side hustles I like range from buying pre-release video game systems (Started with PS3 In 2007), to buying air conditioners in the fall and selling them in the middle of summer. Polishing headlights is a good $50 a car if you got a few simple tools and skills. Cleaning cars is alright cash money too. Try and get repeat business in whatever you do as keeping customer is much easier than attracting new clientele.

Tools

Start collecting high quality tools at a young age. Try to get a rolling, lockable toolbox and put all your prized possessions in there. You should be able to patch a hole in drywall, change a tire, and repair a light fixture. Tools are expensive, so start with high quality names that have a lifetime warranty. Avoid princess auto/ harbour freight unless you need the tool once or twice and plan on returning it. Always keep your purchase receipts in a folder for later use. You might want to sell it and the original bill of sale with the box is always handy.

Books

With all the free libraries popping up in our town I do not buy books anymore. Reading is so beneficial. Paying for books you're going to read once is not. Try this: go to a bookstore and take photos of the books you like, then go home and see if the library has them. If not, ask them to be brought in. Same goes for video games. Most libraries have a very good stock of new video games.

Contracts

Whenever you sign a contract (cell phone, cable plan, extended warranty, work related business), right before you sign, make some comments on the contract regarding how you would like certain things amended. This is your prime negotiation time. Say you are getting a new cell on a two-year contract, the salesperson is making commission and it costs them nothing to modify your plan, so if you want a couple extra gigs data, make sure to ask for it.

Same goes for your cable / internet package. Let's say they will not reduce the monthly rate. You can usually get a couple perks like a few extra channels for free. Say work wants you to sign a contract for certain tasks, or understandings, make sure to get some benefit out of it. It pays to be a shrewd negotiator. Once the sale is complete, you get the taillight warranty. When you can't see their taillights, the warranty is OVER! When you sign a new job offer, make sure to take a copy for yourself, and if you want to negotiate successfully, negotiate in severance pay in case they lay you off. One week for every year is a nice touch. They won't even blink if they need you.

Practice Negotiation Tips

Everything in life is a negotiation. Do not self negotiate away from what you want. In your mind you know what is right for you, so go with your gut and negotiate in your best interests while trying to be fair to others. Negotiation is a game of give and take. Everyone wants to take 51% and give 49%. Be firm. Killing with kindness doesn't work. When people are aware of your presence and that you pull no punches, you can build better trust bonds. If you are a softie all the time people will lie to you more and take advantage of you consciously and subconsciously.

Pay for a Resume Writing Coach

Once you learn the basics of good resume writing, you should keep an updated copy of your resume and email it to yourself, so you always have a copy with you. When you apply for jobs, keep a cover letter template on hand as well that you can tweak for the individual jobs you are applying for. After your application, follow up with a phone call or email to ensure they know you are on point. If you do score an interview, make sure to get the interviewer's contact information. A personalized thank you card from the dollar store may not land you the job, but it can advance you to the short list quickly.

Real Estate

Real estate is the way most people get rich, tax free. In Canada, we are allowed to sell our primary residence tax free if you live in it a year. This is huge. As Kevin Costner said in Wyatt Earp, "A salary has never made a man rich." This is true, your salary is for paying your day-to-day expenses and taking care of bills. With the little money you have left over, you are not going to get rich unless you have ultra low expenses, are a minimalist, or have no kids, regardless of how much money you make.

The most important thing you can do in your early life is purchase some form of real estate with land value. We can build more buildings, higher and higher, but the land underneath is evaporating. Since the pandemic, housing costs in many areas have doubled. Housing typically doubles every 10 years, but sometimes the doubling is often in a tighter timeframe within those 10 years. The same thing happened prior to 2008, housing increased exponentially until the bottom gave way, then shortly afterward housing rocketed back up again. As Warren Buffet says about the stock market, "It's your time in the market, not about timing the market." The same applies to real estate. Think long view and be prepared to run the marathon of life.

Take a vacation

A real one. Not a three-day camping trip with your buddies. I am talking all inclusive where you do not have to think for a week. Not as much culture as you get hiking through the Andes, but your mind will thank you for the rest of the year after you get back to your normal life. After going five times to various all-inclusive, I can say that the bang for the buck is the best in the business. Especially if you can eat and drink your weight in food each day. Pro Tip for hangovers: Prickly Pear juice or capsules. Shut the brain off for a week and watch what happens to your creative side when you return. It explodes.

Screen time

Try to capture how much screen time you are digesting in a typical week and shrink it by 10%. Blue light glasses are a hit now and the research is starting to back it up. Avoid screen time 1-2 hours before bed and avoid checking your cell first thing in the morning while your brain is still in alpha state and impressionable. Try and impression your mind with positive thoughts to instill creativity.

Create a Will

After you die, life goes on for everyone around you. Set up your life before you die so you don't burden anyone when you go. Have a will drawn up and an enduring power of attorney set up once you turn 18. Keep them updated. Have bills and debts on auto pay and clean up any garbage or baggage in your life. Keep your nose clean. Be your own keeper and live like everyday is your last. When you were born, everyone was smiling and you are crying. When you die it should be the opposite.

Watch Your Radiation Levels

Cell phone, airplane, RADON in homes with basements. Be aware. Look for 5G towers, it's uncharted territory.

Drink Tea

Green, black, red, and white tea, doesn't matter, just get it in you! One of my personal favorites from Africa is Rooibos, (Red) Caffeine Free. Which exact tea or brand it makes no difference. Tea has theanine in hit, an amnio acid that helps the brain relax and process information. You can take amnio acids by themselves, but a more natural approach is through tea. Very relaxing, lots of antioxidants, and green tea has been shown to improve fat loss. Organic is best, but not required. I like getting my tea in boxes of 100 from iherb.ca (Canada) or iherb.com for the best value; they pay you to write product reviews.

Debit Cards

Throw away your debit card or keep it in the back of your wallet. Debit cards are the worst. Use a credit card. No interest is charged for the first month and you can often get free points, cash back from purchases, or other perks. My favorite credit card is the Marriot Amex Bonvoy Card. In the past five years I have not paid for a hotel room. Debit cards are more for teenagers starting out in life. They do not have the security features and chargeback options a credit card has, nor the trip insurance, trip cancellation, rental car protection, insurance on new purchases, etc. that are standard for many credit cards.

Read

You're reading right now, so keep that up. Strive for 10 pages a day. Something sustainable. One great leader I follow said they have only read five books but has damn near memorized every word in every book, and in doing so you get a deep meaning and are able to reflect on the true message.

Don't Waste the Weekend

There are 48 hours in a weekend. Try not to waste your weekend "catching up on sleep". Make a goal for every weekend off you have, every year of your life. If you work Monday through Friday, that's 52 goals completed for the year, one for every weekend. That's 520 goals every 10 years. Not every goal is a game changer, but when you add up all the wins you have, the end result could be a life changer.

Get a Labeller or Engraver

Try and label or engrave everything you own that has value to you. For example, if you have a high-end bike or a piece of electronic equipment, scribe your name and phone number into it. If it gets stolen and recovered by the police, you have a high chance of getting it back with your contact information on it. If it shows up in a pawn shop, you can easily get it back. If everyone did this, we would be like Japan where they do not need to lock their bicycles.

Health Insurance

Make sure you always have health insurance and keep your card in your wallet. In Canada you typically pay provincial health premiums. To save your bank, try and get your employer to cover this when you are hired. Elsewhere in the world, fight to make sure you have health care coverage when you get hired at your first job and keep that coverage current. You can often keep coverage going even if you switch jobs by paying a little extra.

Get in the system. Health is wealth. When you are 20 you do not think about it, but when you get older it becomes exponentially more important each year. When travelling, ensure you have health insurance and emergency medical coverage. This may seem like a no brainer, but I remember a story a teacher of mine who often recanted this boring ass story about the time he travelled to the USA and had to whip out his credit card to pay for a splinter removal for his daughter. Back in 1997 the cost was $150 dollars. Today it would probably cost $1000. Thanks Mr. Zee.

And finally...

Learn From others and Share what you know

Communicate efficiently and freely among your peers, friends, and coworkers. Do not hold back. Don't just text on Facebook or Snapchat. Set up a community of minded people where you can share ideas, skills, and beliefs. Start your own tribe if nothing else. Nothing will replace a valuable person. Do not worry about becoming successful. Once you can provide value, success automatically follows. It is hard to become valuable without extracting wisdom from others. Everyone knows something you do not. Try and glean info like a savage. Be savage, ruthless, and unwilling to compromise your values. Be open to love and appreciation for it reflects your true self.